The Emotional Side of Infertility

CHRISSIE JONES

CARTOONS BY JON COOPER

Next Step Publishing 1995
57 Rustlings Road,
Endcliffe,
Sheffield.
S11 7AA
tel 0114 2667674

Printed in England by J.W. Northend Ltd
Clyde Road, Sheffield. S8 OTZ

ISBN 0 9526052 01

British Library Cataloguing in Publication Data. A catalogue record for this book is available from
the British Library.

THE DESIDERATA OF HAPPINESS, which contains the full DESIDERATA, plus other
poems, can be obtained from Souvenir Press, London, or your bookstore.

ACKNOWLEDGEMENT

The production of this book is not the result of one person's work alone. I am grateful for the practical help and enthusiasm of Mike Jones, Sheila Cooke and the counsellors at The Jessop Hospital for Women. I would like to thank them and also those people kind enough to share their feelings during the research for this book.

For making this book possible we gratefully acknowledge the encouragement and financial support given by the following:

Organon

Serono

Sheffield Fertility Centre

Sheffield Health Authority

WellBeing (Sheffield Branch)

Nurture the strength of spririt to shield you in sudden misfortune. But do not distress yourself with imaginings. Many fears are born of fatigue and loneliness. Beyond a wholesome discipline be gentle with yourself.

(Taken from the Desiderata. Max Ehrmann, 1927)

To our Mums and Dads

CONTENTS

Foreword

Anyone who has ever been faced with infertility will recognise the feelings expressed by Chrissie Jones in this book.

Drawing on her own experiences and from others in a similar situation, she describes the frustrations, vulnerability and sadness which beset couples, not merely undergoing investigation and treatment but getting through their daily lives.

She suggests coping strategies with originality, common sense and humour and makes a most valuable contribution to the dilemma of infertility.

Dr. Sheila Cooke
University Department of Obstetrics and Gynaecology
Jessop Hospital for Women
Sheffield
S3 7RE
England

Being without children

Infertility, subfertililty, childlessness, call it what you like; it hurts in many different ways and at many different times. Not being able to have children is more than a medical problem, and whilst more progress is being made on the medical /reproductive side, progress on the emotional side has been slower. There are a few books available which deal with the medical aspects in language that we can all understand, and there are books describing the experiences of infertile couples in a rather lengthy and wordy manner. This book aims to describe the feelings of those undergoing infertility investigations and treatment in a concise and easy-to-read way. Having been through it ourselves and shared experiences with others, it seems there are some common feelings. The intention is to show that the feelings we have are normal and that we should try to deal with these in a positive way which maintains our own dignity. This book is intended for those going through treatment; however, those involved in the treatment and care of people wanting medical help may also find it useful.

The feelings expressed in this book are all genuine ones; some may be those you have experienced, others may not apply to you, but if just a few are meaningful then it has been worthwhile.

It is currently estimated that one in six couples experience infertility at some point. The emotions

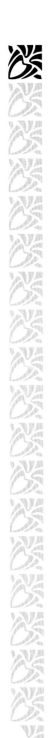

which people experience include anger, frustration, vulnerablity, victimisation, anxiety and many others.

Infertility affects couples and relationships, it is not just an individual concern. The theme expressed here is one of sensitivity to each other's needs as they arise; bearing the pain of infertility alone is a lot harder than sharing it.

The book goes through the natural and sometimes negative thoughts and emotions, with the central theme of putting yourself in control so you can make the right decisions for yourself during this difficult time. Knowledge is power and knowing in advance what you may experience, and that other couples experience similar emotions, is a big step forward in dealing with the situation. There are only a few kinds of life experiences which make us reconsider what is really important and the challenge of infertility is one of them. A common expression heard from couples is, "If you can survive infertility you can survive anything!"

The cartoons have been included because throughout your treatment, it helps to see the occasional funny/bizarre side to what you have to go through.

Keep talking, communication with your partner is important. Don't assume that they will feel exactly the same as you. Seek out the positive. Value yourself and each other.

Good luck and go for it.

I felt so stupid, I burst into tears telling the doctor.

❒ This is often the case, don't worry. Your G.P. should be experienced enough to know that this happens, and should be sympathetic to your situation. It is not easy talking to others about your sex life and plans for children. You get better at it as you realise it is necessary. You can make it easier by breathing slowly, or going with your partner. Talk to people you know and find out who the sympathetic doctors are. Ask to be referred to a specialist if you are not happy with what you are told.

❒ However it helps to be prepared for a long wait. Certainly one thing that takes people by surprise is how long you may have to wait to see various specialists. We hope this does not happen to you, but at least forewarned is forearmed.

❒ We found it a good idea to ask doctors how long we would have to wait before going to the next stage of investigations or treatment. This helps you deal with the wait and if you find yourselves waiting longer you can write or ring.

❒ Unfortunately the Health Service is like any other bureaucracy and sometimes cases may get stuck, so be pro-active, (it will also make you feel better). Don't be afraid to ring the hospital. If your appointment is being delayed because the doctor is on holiday, at least you will know, rather than waiting in the dark.

People keep asking when we are going to start a family.

❐ This is a difficult question yet it is a very common one. You can tell them you don't know but you are having fun practising. This is a light-hearted answer that usually satisfies people.

❐ Or you could try "We are not lucky enough to have them".

❐ On occasions I have simply said I don't want to talk about it, again this is normally respected.

❐ Some have found themselves saying "Oh, we are too busy to be thinking of this", or even "We don't want children". Many of us would find this difficult. Say what you want, to whom you want.

❐ You may be able to think of your own witty response. I personally would never ask anyone this question as it is none of my business.

❐ At different times you may need different answers, be prepared. If you find it difficult to deal with, ask your partner to respond.

Why us?

❏ This is the hardest question to answer and yet it is one that every couple asks/feels at some point. Sometimes we think back and ask what we did wrong but there is little to be gained by thinking in this way. To consider ourselves as "bad people" is nonsense. There is often no reason and these things cannot be explained. It does not help to keep searching for causes that do not exist.

❏ The question we should be asking is what can we do to ensure that we get through this difficult period successfully? Putting ourselves through the agony of working out "Why?" is negative, so generate positive energy and think what can be done to make it easier. The mind does not like pain and will do all it can to resolve the situation. Nobody can promise the childless children. People who say you will get pregnant can give no such guarantee. You may or may not get pregnant.

❏ However one thing that can be guaranteed is that the situation will resolve itself one way or another. Should you not become pregnant, a feeling of acceptance may gradually develop which will allow you to concentrate on other aspects of your life. Time will help with the process of acceptance. The pain you feel now will get less.

❏ It is important to remind yourselves that following infertility treatment, many couples do achieve a pregnancy.

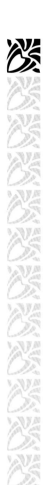

Sometimes I can't bring myself to look at pregnant women or babies in prams.

❒ Even walking down a busy high street can cause pain for a lot of women who are facing the stress of infertility. It seems that once you start trying for a baby, everywhere you go, every magazine you read, every evening you watch television, you come across references to pregnancy and children. It also seems annoyingly easy for some women to get pregnant.

❒ It is possible to avoid going to places where you know there will be lots of children, and sometimes it is easier and more appropriate to do so. Avoiding the stimulus which triggers the emotional pain may be one way of coping. Other strategies include recognising that this happens, and that through treatment, you may one day have a child of your own.

❒ Bear in mind that there will be other people walking down the street, feeling exactly the same, and that some of the babies you see may be the result of assisted conception.

❒ Don't worry that these are strange or irrational thoughts, it is natural to feel envious. These thoughts are commonly held and working through them is part of the healing process. By facing up to your feelings you are on the road to making sense of them, and closer to acceptance of the situation should a pregnancy not arise.

I'm afraid that I won't be able to perform for the sperm test.

❒ Yes this is hard for men (excuse the pun) as they do have to reach a state of sexual arousal in order to produce a sample. At least this is something women do not have to do.

❒ Remember you can take your partner in with you if this may help. Be prepared for pornographic magazines left in the room which may help or offend, depending on your sexual politics.

❒ If this is still difficult for you then ask what else can be done. If you live near the testing laboratory you may be able to take the sample there yourself after having ejaculated at home.

❒ A suggestion for men. Do try to build a close friendship with another man. If you are lucky enough to know someone who is going through similar problems, it can help to share your experiences. Talking to a sympathetic male friend will make it easier to cope.

The emotional side of infertility

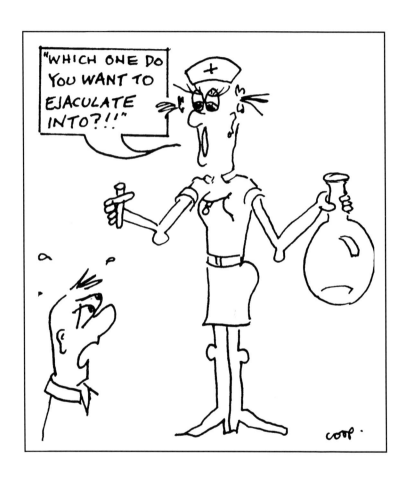

I didn't understand the results of the sperm test.

❒ Putting biological facts in a language that is understandable to us is not easy. Often doctors struggle and can end up using confusing language. Tell them it is not clear.

❒ It might be an idea for you to briefly record your meetings with the doctor, for example, when you saw him/her, what you were told etc. We don't expect the medical profession to remember everything. This really helps you to stay on top of your treatment. You will have a written record of when it started and what was agreed etc.

❒ If you are not sure then go back and ask for more information. Remember, simply giving information is only part of communication; the doctor has to ensure you have understood before he/she can be satisfied.

❒ Read through a medical book, perhaps talk to your G.P., but be careful about asking a "medical friend/relative"; often they may not have the level of knowledge required to help and may wrongly advise you.

My friend is pregnant, I feel so jealous.

❏ This is natural. You would be a saint if you did not feel like this. Think carefully before sharing the experience of childlessness. A woman who is going through the joys of pregnancy may not be the best one to talk to.

❏ You do not have to tell your friend. Some of us found that after the birth of the baby the feelings of jealousy disappeared, as the pleasure of seeing the baby reminded us that jealousy is a negative emotion. Some of us felt more jealous of pregnant women than those with babies, it is different for everyone.

❏ However, if the relationship is a close one you may feel it is appropriate to tell her. Some of us found it easier to talk to people who had experienced a loss of some sort, whether it be a death, miscarriage or divorce.

❏ Try to see your friend as different. You can be happy for her and sad for yourself at the same time, they are not exclusive emotions.

❏ Talk to your partner, he/she can help you through these times.

I feel so lonely.

❏ When we are afraid and lonely we can easily become isolated and can be prone to depression, so it really does help to keep active. Involving yourself in the lives of others may stop you getting too self-centered.

❏ It is true that gender plays a part in how we deal with problems, and sometimes we can benefit from the coping strategies adopted by the other gender. Men often keep their feelings to themselves and kid themselves that the problem will go away, simply by ignoring it and keeping active. Women may sometimes torture themselves by going over the problem. So, men, it may help to talk, and women, it may help to do things with friends. You don't have to talk about it all the time, in fact some people may get frustrated. You must keep other interests even when it seems like nothing is going to happen.

❏ Think about how you could share these feelings. You need to remember, that while you have given a lot of thought to this, it may be new to your family. Don't expect them to understand straight away. Give them time, perhaps plan a walk together. You could consider a support group. There are benefits to joining a local or national support group. You can get help, advice and perhaps most importantly, an opportunity to talk to others going through the same experience.

❏ Keep an interest in other issues. You will have more to offer a child. Reading up on baby care may be too much, but the more interests you have the better, and the more sane you will remain!

The emotional side of infertility

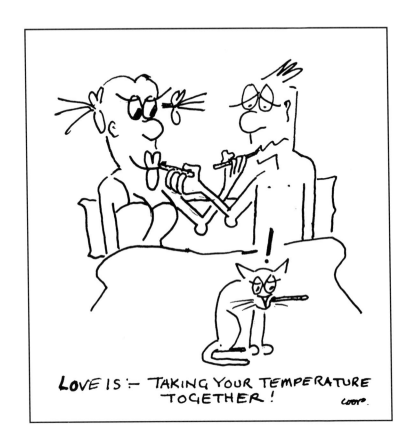

LOVE IS :- TAKING YOUR TEMPERATURE TOGETHER !

I am sick of charting, why does it have to be the woman?

❒ Get your partner to record his temperature every morning, at least then, he will have an idea of what it's like. You could ask him to read your temperature and plot it on the chart, but make sure you both know what you're doing.

❒ Showing him the charts gets him interested, and allows him to demonstrate to you that he does care. Men often find it easier to do things, (O.K. it's a bit sexist!). You may be pleasantly surprised to find that your partner wants to get practically involved. Some men said they felt helpless and unable to support their partners as much as they would have liked throughout the treatment. Here is a way they can show that they care as much as you do. Just as when a new baby arrives, encouraging Dad to share in the responsibility for looking after the baby, makes him feel included.

❒ Ask him (or get him) to make you a cup of tea while you go through your three minute ritual every morning. This will give both of you a routine, and the two of you get to have a drink together and have a good start to the day.

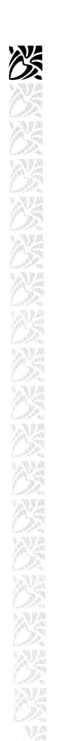

Starting the day off doing temperature charts is horrible.

❏ Yes, but at least it reminds you that you are doing something useful every day, you are in control and this information will help you and the medical staff. When we are under pressure it's hard to be rational about doing things we don't like, but it is useful, try to accept it.

❏ It gets easier, honest. In fact, it helps to show if you are under the weather with 'flu or whatever. However, it is a pain taking everything with you on holiday, at a time when you perhaps need a break from the worry of infertility. Check with your medical team for how long you have to do it, it may be a shorter time than you think.

❏ Again, keep reminding yourself that by doing this you are helping to resolve the problem. Every day brings you closer to a solution. The more information you can provide for the medical team, the more they can plan the best treatment (and the timing of it) for you. There is nothing intrinsically unpleasant about this routine, it is how you perceive it. Do see it as an action which means you are starting the day off actively working towards conception.

I cry unexpectedly.

❏ This is a positive release of feelings that have built up over a stressful period. Physiologically, crying can and does make us feel better. Don't be hard on yourself. For many of us it is a safe way of combating the pain, and again was found to be very common.

❏ Try to identify the reasons why you are crying - out of desperation, self pity, frustration, loneliness? You can then begin to tell your partner and he/she can make you feel better, and can comfort you through this difficult time. It might help to discuss these feelings with a counsellor or a close friend. It can be embarrassing if you are crying in public places. Some of us found it helpful to focus on a happy experience to temporarily blot out these feelings, until we were in a place where we could cry safely.

❏ What is really making you cry? Are you tired, do you need a break, is it the time of the month? If you think about the reason you can then do something about solving it.

❏ Remember many of us spend years suffering the monthly tension of waiting to see if a pregnancy has taken place, then coping with the disappointment and sadness if it has not. Similarly the frustration of waiting for the results of investigations or treatment is cumulative and like most forms of stress, it needs an outlet. Be gentle with yourself.

Sex is awful, it's so mechanical.

❏ Do you mean sex for reproduction? It may help to see this as separate from sex for pleasure and enjoyment. Most animals have sex solely for reproduction, but we humans can experience it for pleasure. Try to maintain the pleasure aspects at other times.

❏ There will be times in the month when it would be a good idea to make love, but sometimes you or your partner may not feel like it. Which is more important, your self-esteem or trying? The answer may be different every month. Don't force it.

❏ Do find time to compliment each other , find time to support each other. What could you do to help if it doesn't feel right? Soft music, baby oil........

❏ Do be gentle on yourselves. If you are under a lot of pressure, it's natural that your sex life may suffer, but it is very likely to be temporary. Be compassionate with one another. Think back to the fun you had, it will come again.

The emotional side of infertility

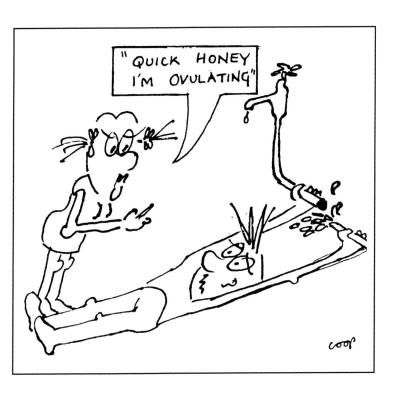

I can't get an erection any more.

❏ Again this is often more common than you think and is a natural response to having to "perform". Remember you have had them before and it's likely you will get them again.

❏ Talk to your partner (but not when you are in bed) about why you feel this way. She needs to support you now as you have supported her.

❏ What kinds of experiences turn you on? See if you can try something you both like.

❏ If it continues, you could talk to your G.P. or even a friend. This can be a spin off from infertility because you learn to talk more openly with others. In this way you can get support and get in touch with your feelings.

❏ For men who have infertility problems, it is easy to transfer the physical failure to produce healthy motile sperm into a psychological feeling of failure. The two are separate and you are not a failure.

Every month I get so depressed, my body won't do what I want.

❏ Your body is not under your conscious control. This book is about concentrating on what you can control, so don't blame yourself.

❏ Think of your body as a treasure. It really is an amazing system, it will help you, so don't blame it.

❏ When did you last pamper your body? It's working hard for you so go on, treat yourself.

❏ It's a strange fact about human beings that when something goes wrong we often seek to blame something or someone, yet this is not always the best way of reacting. Think positively not about what you can't do, but about what you can do.

❏ However, if you do feel down now and again, think of the good things you can do and the successes you have achieved. We all need our good points reaffirming now and again. This is where you can help your partner, who may also need his/her self image reinforced.

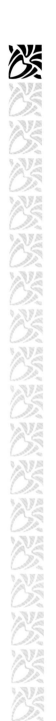

I feel my partner won't love me because I am infertile.

❐ Love is a very powerful emotion and whilst it is easy to say that "true love" can survive anything, in reality it is not always that easy. Let your partner know how you feel. It's good to remind yourselves why you love each other.

❐ The problem of infertility does not change the relationship between you, but it puts it under the microscope and any weaknesses are shown. In reality a lot of us found that it deepened our love, as we battled through it together. So good luck.

❐ It is important that you discuss things clearly together before you decide on the course of treatment you want. For example, if you are considering donor sperm/eggs it is essential you both understand and agree wholeheartedly with the treatment.

❐ Unfortunately infertility can evoke feelings of guilt. Whilst this can be a natural reaction, it is unhelpful in the long run. Self-respect is important and positive, and by loving yourself you make it easier for your partner to love you.

I heard a man at work talking about firing blanks.

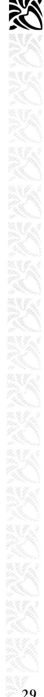

❏ People don't realise that men too can be hurt by such passing remarks, and it is often difficult to know what to do, when you are angered by such comments. Modern society does not make it easy for men to open up, and unfortunately some see a show of feelings as unmanly.

❏ Don't get too down-hearted by such throw away comments. Keep reminding yourself that whilst you are not in control of your body you can still control the way you see yourself.

❏ You have a number of options, depending on the situation and how you feel at the time. You could walk away and reassure yourself that you are no less of a man because of this. Don't blame yourself for what you cannot help. We don't blame or laugh at people who cope with medical conditions such as diabetes; infertiltity is no different.

❏ If you are feeling confident you could challenge his comments by questioning whether a man's masculinity is purely linked to reproduction. If you decide to use donor sperm, being a loving father to a child every day is much more important than being simply the sperm provider.

❏ Recent research has shown that infertile fathers are more involved with their children (and much more sensitive than the bloke you over heard!). Source: Adoption UK, no. 71, November 1994 page 39.

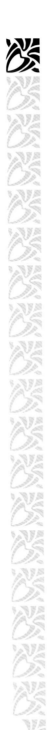

My periods have gone haywire.

❏ Did you know that emotional factors can affect your menstrual cycle? Your cycle may shorten or lengthen because of the stress you are experiencing. Don't worry, think positively. The length of the cycle may have changed but it is still likely you are ovulating.

❏ This is more common than perhaps you think. One woman was regular for over 15 years but as soon as the visit to hospital for treatment started, her cycle went haywire. The medical staff will be able to support you, as this is commonly experienced.

❏ Similarly if you are under stress, say from bereavement, your periods may become irregular. Again infertility teaches us that we should not take anything for granted.

❏ Irregular periods are quite common. Did you know that ovulation prediction kits are available? You can buy these from the clinic or a chemist. They are quite expensive, however they will give you a better idea of when you are about to ovulate, unlike the temperature charts which really give you an indication of when you have ovulated.

It's useless, all the semen comes out.

❏ Whilst the semen does inevitably come out of the vagina following ejaculation, sufficient sperm for fertilisation are already in the neck of the womb and have started their journey towards the egg, therefore you do not need to worry. Remember it only takes "one little blighter" to get through.

❏ Don't be afraid to ask for practical advice. The medical team are there to help you and they have experienced a whole range of questions and queries. Going through infertility investigations makes you more ready to ask for medical advice generally, as any natural shyness usually disappears fairly quickly.

❏ A common belief is that there are certain positions to adopt during and after sexual intercourse which will improve your chances of conception. Medical thinking now informs us that this is not the case. This is good news for all of us, except contortionists!

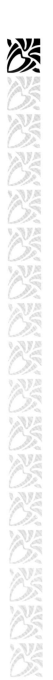

Different doctors interpret results differently.

❒ This is confusing. We sometimes expect doctors to be like parents, always knowing the answers. In reality a doctor's role is more difficult. They have to assess your case and make decisions about what constitutes the best treatment for you.

❒ The results of your tests are facts but these need to be interpreted, and different doctors may give you different interpretations. It may help to ask for the best and worst interpretations. Doctors are there to help you. They can discuss the implications of your results and suggest which treatment offers you the best chance of a pregnancy.

❒ When you are awaiting the results of tests you are often emotional and anxious. It is easy to hear only the bad news, or forget some of what the doctor has said. Sometimes, no matter how carefully doctors try to tell us about infertility when the news is broken, you are in a state of shock, and when they say 'Have you got any questions?' your mind goes blank. It may be an idea to have possible questions worked out in advance. Don't be afraid to ring up later if you are unsure of something. There may not be anyone available to help there and then, but a good hospital will always follow up such requests.

The emotional side of infertility

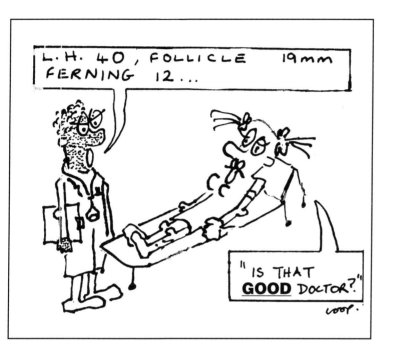

I am afraid of a laparoscopy (or other such treatment).

❐ Why are you afraid? You are allowing something to be done which will help you plan the next stage. See it as a positive step.

❐ The full medical team will be able to help you. They are experienced and very competent.

❐ Can your partner be around to help before and after? Tell him what you would like. If you don't have it done you won't find out if there is a problem. Which will be the more difficult to deal with?

❐ Whatever procedure is being carried out, find out what will be involved. Ask the doctors, although sometimes the nurses are better at explaining what this will be like. This should help you prepare. Be careful of horror stories from other patients who have had the same treatment, they may have a different pain threshold to you.

❐ Finally on a personal note, none of the treatment I experienced was particularly painful, perhaps only mild discomfort, and that included a hysterosalpingogram (see glossary) and a laparoscopy.

The emotional side of infertility

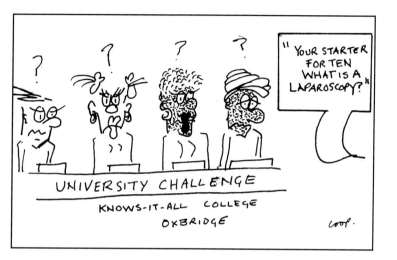

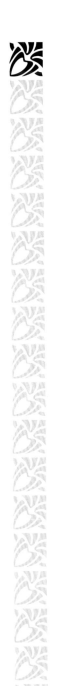

I have blocked tubes, I can't believe it.

❐ It takes time for any news to sink in and it's hoped the information was broken to you in a sensitive way. There are certain stages we go through when we get bad news and although it may seem like the end of the world, the medical profession can do a lot more to help these days.

❐ See this as a step forward. You have been told something which means the medical team can now give you options to consider and all the time you are moving forward in the matter. You now have information which can help you make decisions.

❐ Another tip is ,'Don't rush yourselves'. You have been given news which has saddened you, but humans are amazingly resourceful and in time the shock will lessen, and you will feel better.

❐ Like most medical problems there are degrees of blockage and often more than one option is available. Make sure you hear and understand what the doctor meant, as sometimes when we receive bad news we only hear the negative side and latch onto certain words. When we are emotionally upset then our memory is often selective.

I can't decide whether to go for I.V.F. or not.

❏ Making decisions about infertility treatments is like any other major life choice. For a start, one partner may want to go for I.V.F. or other such treatment and may put presssure on the other when they are not ready. Nobody can make the decision for you. We usually make these decisions based on a combination of heart and head. It goes without saying that you must both agree on the course of action. If you are undecided then collect information about the treatment processes, discuss these with your doctor, counsellor, nurse. It may be an idea to talk with couples for whom it has been successful and with those for whom it has not, so you can learn from their experiences.

❏ To help you make the decision some "fors" and "againsts" are suggested. For: you may get a pregnancy; you may find out what is causing the infertility, and thus can plan ahead; you will be comforted by the fact that you tried; the more couples try, the more the techniques can be improved. Against: the stress of treatment and the possibility of the treatment not working may be too difficult to bear; the cost of treatment may be prohibitive; finding out that there is a specific problem may be too much for some and thus they avoid the opportunity of finding out; some may be put off by the physical side of the treatment. Although you will come to your own decision, it may help to write your thoughts down and then come back to them a week later and see if there are any changes. Take time if you need it. You can come back to treatment at a later date if you are not ready now.

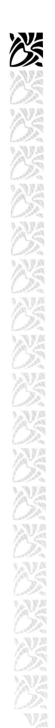

The treatment is so expensive, we can't afford it.

❏ Some Health Authorities are now prepared to pay for In Vitro Fertilisation and Donor Insemination but this may mean going on to a long waiting list. Eligibility for funding can also be strict e.g. age of the woman, previous children. It is always helpful to compare the criteria used by different Authorities, as they do vary. In one case a couple actually moved house, in order to qualify for treatment with a neighbouring Authority!

❏ We need to highlight the inadequate and unequal funding of infertility treatment. For some this means the treatment is totally inaccessible. Health Authorities need to be continually reminded that this is unacceptable. More open discussion of this situation will help to improve awareness of this issue.

❏ The National Infertility Awareness Campaign (NIAC) has information on the services provided within each Health Authority. Should you want to take an active part in campaigning for more infertility treatment on the NHS, you should contact NIAC on 0800 716345 for a free information pack containing details of local and national events such as their "Focus Week" with advice on how to write to your MP and Health Authority.

❏ If you have to pay, it is worth finding out exactly how much. Does the price quoted include cost of drugs? Does the cost of a laparoscopy include the surgeon's fee, the anaesthetist's fee and hospital accommodation? If you do have private medical insurance, make sure you understand what it offers.

I can't tell my Mum or Dad.

❏ It is very difficult to tell our parents. They may have hopes, even expectations of grandchildren and so may feel a combination of loss, sadness and anger. Also for us there may be a sense that we have let the family side down. Infertiltity and guilt often go hand in hand. These are irrational and unhelpful ways of viewing the situation, yet these sorts of reasons make us reluctant to tell our parents. Like you, they need time to come to terms with the news, so don't expect a necessarily sympathetic response straight away. It's more likely they will go through in a slightly different way some of the stages you have gone through. Reflect upon the numbness you may have experienced when you were first told, this may help you to appreciate how they feel now.

❏ People who have had children often cannot offer advice to those without children, and don't forget this can apply to parents too.

❏ Some of you may decide not to tell your parents, whilst others will. The key principle is that it is your body, your life, your information. If you do decide to tell, consider whether you want your partner there to help break the news. Pick the moment carefully, a busy family gathering is less appropriate than a quiet country walk.

I don't want to go to the christening.

❏ These are particularly painful times as they bring all our feelings to the fore. There is no easy solution, but the following suggestions may help. (Statistically you are not likely to be the only couple who are facing or have faced this problem at the Christening.)

❏ Could you just go to the church? If you arrive late and leave early people will be too busy to notice your absence.

❏ Ask another friend or family member in advance to keep an eye on you and help you out, if it appears that you are going to get upset. If someone asks that dreaded question "do you have children?" they can be ready to step in and change the subject.

❏ It's up to you to accept or reject the invitation. You could tell your friend that it is too difficult for you or simply phone up on the day with a headache. Everybody will be busy on the day and unlikely to miss you.

The emotional side of infertility.

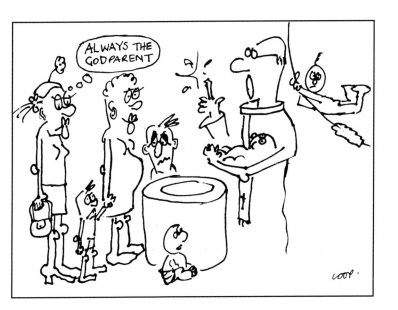

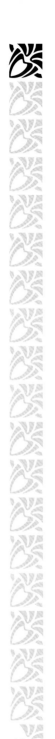

I have to take time off work, I can't tell my boss why.

❑ So what, they don't have to know. Sometimes white lies protect us. They do not have a right to know everything about us. Would it help if you told them? Do you want them asking how it's going all the time? Can they be relied upon to keep confidences? Have you trusted them before? In childhood we learn that telling lies is wrong, but sometimes it is necessary, so don't feel guilty. Are they in a position to understand? How did they deal with other employees who experienced personal problems? If they were genuinely supportive then you may want to tell them, and the more infertility becomes something we can openly talk about the better. One of us had a boss who had been through infertility and gone on to adopt, so it was easier to talk to her. Every time we talk about infertility we make it easier for future couples to discuss. Unfortunately the problem of infertility is here to stay.

❑ There are still taboos attached to infertility. If your kidneys didn't work properly and you needed time off work you wouldn't dream of not telling your boss, but if you have a problem with your reproductive organs then it is not considered a topic for discussion. ONLY, if you feel strong enough should you tell your boss. It is good to discuss and try to change people's misconceptions about infertility, but you must be in control. It might help to take someone in with you. Unfortunately when women start talking about babies some bosses can become quite sexist. Make up your own mind as to what you want to do.

I hate lying at work, I've had so many fake 'flu attacks.

❏ Yes, thinking of reasons why you cannot be at work is not easy; even if your boss knows, you don't want every one knowing your business. Some hospitals can arrange for treatment at a time which is convenient for you. However should you need excuses good examples of reasons why you are not at work could include: a broken tooth which necessitates immediate treatment, 'flu, food poisoning, being locked out, witnessing a road accident! Use your imagination. You decide what is the best to tell others. Don't be too hard on yourself. In the history of employment people have done much worse.

❏ It is not easy getting time off work when you need it. Some people may have to travel quite a way for treatment, but ask yourself: is it worth it? If you have given good service then you deserve a little licence.

❏ If you have told your boss, fine, but you do not have to tell everyone. To be honest, there is a mixture of what works best. If you don't tell people where you are going then you don't get asked lots of difficult questions, but you don't get any support if you need it. Again the message is keep yourself in control.

❏ It may help to have friends who can cover for you and help you through tricky times. They are worth their weight in gold!

Waiting lists are so long, I feel like nobody cares.

❒ Yes, this may be the case, infertility treatment may have a low priority, but you cannot control this, so concentrate on what you can control. You could write a few letters to the hospital and your local M.P. and watch out for events like National Infertility Awareness Week.

❒ Does the hospital have a support group where you could meet others? Hospitals that care usually provide this or can give you an address.

❒ Your friends care about you. It's up to you whom you choose to talk to. Talk to those you know will be supportive. Many of us found that, once we started talking about infertility, other people had experienced it in some form. It may have taken a long time for them to conceive or for themselves to have been conceived. They may have adopted, or be adopted, or have given a child up for adoption. Honestly, it is a lot more common than you think.

❒ People often try to give you advice, fine, but it is up to you if you decide to take it or not. Tell whom you want, when you want.

My partner is more upset than I am.

❐ Often one partner may experience more pain than the other. This is often the woman who in our society is seen as the prime carer. Some believe that women experience more maternal feelings than men. Whatever the cause, whether it is genetic or cultural, in our society reproduction is linked more strongly with women than men.

❐ This is a time when you can help your partner. Think what you can do to improve the situation? Reassurance of your love is important. If you can think of something which will make him/her feel better, try to arrange it.

❐ Do take care of your partner. Childlessness hurts and it is natural to cry, but depression is another matter, so keep a gentle and watchful eye on them. Professional advice is always available via your G.P.

❐ When you are upset you may think you are bearing the brunt of childlessness yourself. Your partner might feel the same but doesn't show it as much. It really does help to let your partner know how you feel.

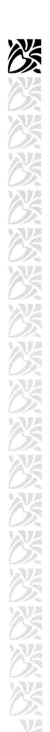

My partner doesn't seem to be bothered.

❏ Some of us deal with problems in different ways. Some are like ostriches, and think if they leave something alone it will go away. There are some advantages to this approach, but psychologically it is very difficult to deny these feelings over a long time. We need to deal with them but at our own pace and when we are ready.

❏ Sometimes people need more encouragement to show their feelings. Can you help them? Can you show and reassure them that you love them? Can you make it clear to them that you want to know how they feel? ●

❏ This is often the way men deal with problems especially those of an emotional nature, so they may need more time. They receive messages that it is unmanly to talk about feelings from an early age, so give them time.

❏ Share the appointment making and treatment practices so that they are familiar with what happens. Try to get them to do their fair share; making a baby needs two people which ever means you use.

❏ It is isolating if you think that you are going through this on your own, especially if your partner is busy with other jobs. Try to remind them that time is passing and the chance of success is reduced as one gets older.

I hate not being in control.

❐ For some women there is the particular frustration of not being able to control what happens. This is especially so for those who have control in other aspects of their lives, for example at work, or in relationships. Many expressed the frustrations of being controlled by drugs, doctors' waiting lists, the necessity of having intercourse at certain times of the month, and the invasive nature of tests etc.

❐ It may help to try to think beyond these feelings. Aim to develop a sort of "que sera, sera" attitude and concentrate on those things you can exert influence over. For example we know it is silly to worry about the weather, we recognise that it is beyond our control and we have learned to accept that some days it may rain.

❐ It is often the case that infertility turns previously sane and emotionally stable adults into emotionally fractious people. Sometimes, we find ourselves out of control of our feelings, for example we may cry unexpectedly, or fly off the handle at the smallest thing. It may help to plan for periods of anxiety; cut out stressful activities, try to maintain control in appointments with doctors, e.g. have your questions ready. As we mature into adulthood we learn to control our emotions, sometimes even feigning them. Remember that every couple you see going to the fertility clinic is going through the same emotions as you, no matter how outwardly confident or self-assured they may appear.

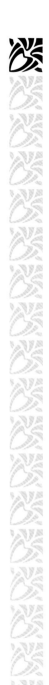

I am scared people will see me as a failure or pity me.

❐ They might, that is their problem. We all assume that we are fertile and if we find out we are not then it is a bit of a surprise to say the least, but you can't help it, and you are not a failure.

❐ Failures are people who do not do what they could and you are doing everything you can to help the situation. By following medical advice as to how to increase your chances of fertility, for example watching your consumption of alcohol or losing weight etc, means you are giving yourself the best chances of conception. Anything else is beyond your control.

❐ However, if you do feel down now and again then think of the good things that you can do, the successes you have achieved. We all need our good points reaffirming now and again. You can improve your partner's self-esteem by emphasising his/her achievements.

❐ People are always willing to give advice if they think they can help. Again, it's up to you if you decide to take it. Having a strong sense of self worth is important now, how others see you really is a lesser concern.

I hate Christmas, I have to pretend I am O.K.

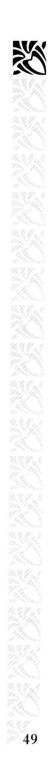

❐ Christmas is all about families and when we don't have the family we want it hurts perhaps more than at any other time of year, so prepare yourself in advance.

❐ It's also true that the birth of Jesus reminds us all of birth and children. For some of us it brought back happy childhood memories of our own family Christmases. We had hoped that we could share the much loved family traditions with our own children.

❐ Find people who can be sympathetic at this time. You can let them know that it is a difficult time for you. Most people want to help if they know your situation, but often do not know the best way of going about it. Telling them lets them know. Alternatively, you may want a quiet time away from everyone. You can do this. Go to a hotel by the seaside if you fancy it.

❐ Some of us found that visualisation helps. Rather than thinking negatively of the sad, childless Christmases, think of the happy times you have had. Visualise yourself in a situation in which you feel relaxed and unstressed.

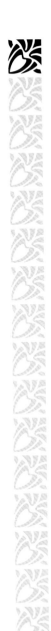

I cry when I see children being hurt on television.

❒ This is a normal reaction. We often wonder how people can be cruel to children, however it is not much use distressing yourself further. Switch it off if it upsets you. (Unless you are a real glutton for punishment, avoid watching 'Children in Need'!)

❒ Life at this time can be unfair. Here are you wanting to have and care for children, and yet some people are unable to care for their own children, sometimes causing senseless pain to their offspring. Use this time positively to think and discuss with your partner how you would cope with a demanding child or difficult behaviour. You can plan ahead together.

❒ Think about the children you know in your life, perhaps nephews, nieces, children of friends and neighbours; what can you do to help them enjoy life? The role provided by aunts, uncles, family and friends is often underestimated. Many of us have happy memories of times spent with such people, when perhaps on occasions our parents seemed too busy for us. They were special for us. People without children of their own are important for all children. There is an African proverb which succintly sums this up. "It takes a whole community to raise a child".

Our marriage is suffering.

❒ This is common, particularly if only one partner has been diagnosed as being infertile. It is natural to think about what might have been with another partner. We often try to blame the other person, but this gets us nowhere. The infertile person cannot control the infertility and therefore cannot be blamed.

❒ You have made a commitment to your partner so think about the strategies you can use to help. Be clear, tell your partner what you would like him/her to do. Make a list of how you can help each other.

❒ If you have been through difficult times before, what things helped you then? Can you use these now? Would it help to talk to Relate? This is a confidential service which some find helpful.

❒ Sometimes with infertility we place demands upon our partner which are too great for any one person to bear. Sometimes your partner may not be the best person to give help as they may be struggling themselves. Treat yourselves. You are both special. Do something you enjoy.

The past is getting me down.

❏ Nowadays there may be a variety of scenarios for which this statement is true. As relationships are increasingly breaking down and people re-marry, the "reconstituted family" becomes more common, and it may be the case that your partner has had children in a previous relationship. This can compound your feeling of failure and heighten a sense of jealousy. Also in more than one case I came across couples where one partner had not told the other that they had had a vasectomy, or that they knew they would have difficulties conceiving. This is unfair and very hard to deal with. We all have a right to know such information. Not only might the person be devastated by this news, but the fact that their partner had lied to them, would make it doubly hard to live with. For some the case may be one of abortion, or giving a child up for adoption. It is easy to understand how these actions now seem regrettable, but at the time appeared to be for the best.

❏ Don't dwell on the past too much, recognise that what's done is done. Your partner is now with you, and your partner loves you. It is inevitable that you will experience some negative emotions, perhaps a sense of regret, but try to live from where you are now and look to the future. Do communicate these feelings, share this challenge together and never under-estimate the .power of a hug to make you feel better. Don't wear yourself out going over the past, you need all your energy to deal with the challenge of infertility.

I look at our wedding pictures and feel sad.

❏ Our society takes fertility for granted. It is assumed that when we get married we will automatically have children, however we know that this is not the case. Remember you got married for better or worse. Better times will come.

❏ Remember you feel sad not because you got married to your partner but because you are finding it difficult to have children. You may not be married but you still have a strong commitment to each other, so as you go through difficult times together and survive together, your relationship will become deeper and closer.

❏ For some the pain and difficulty may be too great and divisions may set in. In a way it might be better to find out before you have children that dealing with any crisis is too much for you both. Infertility can place a big strain on a relationship so don't give up too soon. There is a sense of achievement. "Surviving infertility means you can survive anything" was a response from one couple.

❏ It's likely you never expected that there would be difficulties in conceiving and this naturally comes as a shock. If we are able to talk to younger people in a responsible way about infertility we make it slightly easier for successive generations to come to terms with it.

The pain of infertility does not get any easier.

❏ No, but you can get better at dealing with it and over time you will develop your own strategies for coping. We found these to include laughing sessions, regular talking and listening sessions, monitoring the good things we have, sharing in the care of nieces and nephews, to name but a few. Nothing can really substitute for having children, but some things can help to make it better.

❏ Don't put yourself under any unnecessary stress and avoid situations which you don't have to go through, for example, christenings. Keep yourself in control. Identify the occasions which are most difficult to deal with and see if you can do anything to avoid these, or plan how you can handle them. Although the pain doesn't get any less, listening to people who have lived with infertility for a long time, it is clear that you are more able to cope with situations which previously would have upset you. Every couple finds ways which are right for them, including confrontation and avoidance. It's important to realise that you may use different ways at different times.

❏ Some of us noticed seasonal variations. It is natural to feel lower in winter. The lack of sunshine can affect some people particularly badly. Plan for this and have treats to look forward to during this colder spell. Look over your summer photos, or plan that summer break for the following year.

The emotional side of infertility

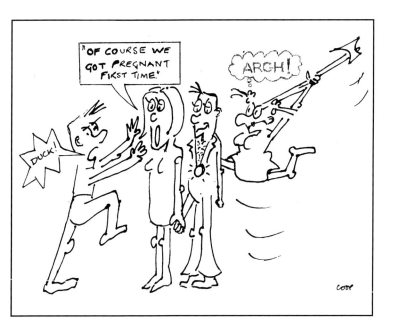

I am sick of folk telling me "don't worry, it will be O.K."

❒ This is very common and often painful to hear. People who have not been through this really cannot understand how distressing it can be, and how easily it can take over the whole of your life. You cannot stop yourself from thinking about it, day in day out.

❒ Latterly I got quite off-hand with people who made this remark and asked them if they would be able to stop worrying if a loved one was diagnosed as having cancer. This worked.

❒ However, there is a difference between sitting at home feeling sorry for yourself and getting busy and doing things. Aerobic exercise, for example swimming, naturally relaxes the body by releasing endorphins which will have a calming effect on your emotional state.

❒ It may be the case that if you are paying for treatment you may not be able to afford a holiday, but at least try to do something you like, you do deserve it. Have you had a tickling fight with your partner? Have you had a really good laugh? It will make you feel better. Infertility is pretty grim, and without a sense of humour it's even worse.

I have thought of sleeping with someone else.

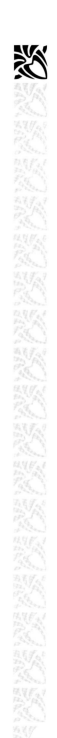

❏ Haven't we all at some point? No, being serious, this seems a simple way out if the infertility is on the male side and there is no harm in thinking about it. However, in reality, this is not a good idea and would only complicate matters. We just wanted to reassure you that this is another common reaction, so don't feel you are letting the side down with these thoughts. It is much better to discuss with your doctors the next course of action.

❏ When children are created using donor sperm/eggs, there are issues which need to be thrashed out. The hospital will have to provide you with counselling before you embark on this treatment. You will have plenty of opportunities to think about the consequences and the law protects you. This is a much safer way of obtaining donor sperm.

❏ It's natural, no matter how close you are to your partner, you always have some thoughts which are better left unsaid. For some it may be appropriate to see the counsellor alone. You will have the chance to discuss these feelings, recognising you may have different needs to your partner. It may be worth trying to arrange an apppointment with an independent counsellor as often friends and family may be emotionally too close to both of you and of course they cannot offer trained specialist couselling. You may like to take advantage of the confidential 24 hour telephone service offered by self help groups e.g. "Child" and "Issue". See page 76 for details.

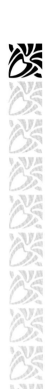

I don't want to see certain friends any more.

❏ It is often the case that infertility can change our relationships with some friends. You may lose contact with some because you don't feel you can talk to them or they feel uneasy in your company. They may feel they can't say anything which might upset you and this starts to put a strain on the relationship. Decide whether the costs outweigh the benefits of continuing the relationship. It's true that in times of crisis, you do find out who your real friends are.

❏ You can tell people you don't want to talk about it or you can decide to share your feelings; remember they are probably thinking about your situation.

❏ It is a fact of life that we make new friends and leave old ones behind. It is also likely that you will meet new people through the hospital etc. who have been in similar situations and perhaps are more understanding. New relationships may develop.

❏ One couple who had discussed their infertility with many of their friends, chose not to tell others in order to have a break from questions from well meaning people. Again you decide whatever you feel most comfortable with.

People have stopped talking about it since we told them.

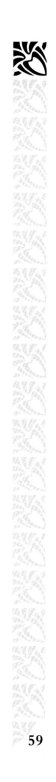

❏ Don't worry, many of us found this was the case and there are a variety of reasons why people may do this. For example my Mum stopped talking to us about it, an attitude we initially interpreted as a little uncaring. When we did mention it, she said she didn't want to upset us, but she would happily listen/help if we wanted her to. When couples are undergoing investigations there is a tendency to continuosly worry that someone may just be about to ask about children, treatment, etc; at an inappropriate time. Some friends and family sense this and therefore avoid the topic. Others may assume that as you have not raised the subject you have given up with treatment.

❏ It's a sad fact that some people do not like talking about difficult things. Others simply know that incessant questions understandably upset you and thus avoid them, knowing that if there is good news you will soon share it. People are different and we need to recognise this. Keep friends informed when it seems appropriate.

❏ It also depends where you meet. Talking about not being able to have children is not really pub talk.

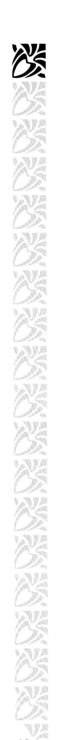

We are in a "catch 22", the more treatments we have the more desperate we become.

❏ New treatments are developing all the time and the results with existing ones are improving too, offering better chances of pregnancy. However in the 1940s and '50s, there was little help available for couples. One woman who had blocked tubes said she obviously regretted not being able to have children, but she believes in some respects the lack of treatments available, meant she faced up to infertility sooner. She was spared the incessant desire to try just one more time, thus laying herself open to more bitter disappointment. There is something to consider here. Knowing when to start, and when to stop treatment, is part of keeping yourself in control. It is your life.

❏ It is difficult to know when to stop treatment, and it is hoped that this is not a decision you have to make (i.e. the treatment works and you get pregnant). However, it can be distressing watching your partner invest so much energy that they become tired and unable to make decisions. It may be useful to talk to your doctor or counsellor, who may be able to help you make your decision to stop, or even have a break.

❏ When I asked a nurse how many cycles we should try, she advised we shouldn't put a limit on it, but rather, see how we felt each time. We did, and I think you know when you have reached your emotional limit yourselves.

Now we have stopped treatment, it feels so strange.

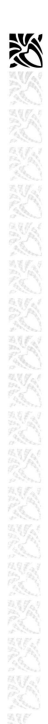

❐ If the treatment is successful, then brilliant, if it isn't, you need time to adjust. It may help to mark the end of this era in your life with some sort of event, a meal to treat yourselves. See it as a positive end to that part of your life. You will always be comforted by the fact that you tried.

❐ Listening to older couples who are childless, it seems that the pain of infertility doesn't necessarily get any less, but you certainly develop more effective coping strategies and learn to avoid those situations, which you know instinctively, will trigger off unhappy feelings.

❐ One couple said, that at at least as you get older, people stop asking you when you are going to have children. It is possible to come through this period in your lives together and with a greater understanding of what you want. Enjoy the time together.

❐ Some of us will choose not to return to treatment. Others will recognise they need a break and may plan to restart when they feel ready. It's a personal decision for each couple.

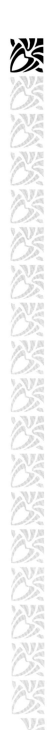

I wish I hadn't married my partner, things would have been different.

❐ Unfortunately this is a genuine thought for some, the kind of thing that may get shouted out in an argument, or secretly felt in a quiet moment. If it is your partner who has been diagnosed as being infertile, then it's tempting to think how your life would have differed if you had married another.

❐ The reality of life is that we have to deal with what we are faced with, the present has to be addressed squarely. People who live in the past seldom reach happiness.

❐ Try to move on and see how you can face this together, remember infertility affects the two of you, it is a shared concern. It is difficult to know which is the more distressing, finding you are infertile or that you cannot have children with your partner. Each brings its own feelings of frustration and intense disappointment. Take the first step and share your feelings.

❐ Many couples do survive this time in their lives and find their relationship grows, perseverance is worth the reward. I did encounter people whose relationship had irretrievably broken down because of the strain of infertility, and this too is understandable. Work out what is best for you, concentrate on your strengths as a couple. There is no need to rush it.

Sometimes I feel like I have lost a child I never had.

❐ Following the initial distress of not achieving a pregnancy, there is more to face, namely the realisation that a greater loss has taken place. This loss is more than not being able to give birth to a baby, it is the loss of a child, a teenager, an adult child, and all the accompanying pleasures that children bring. It is a common feeling which some have likened to the psychological experience of a miscarriage or even the death of a child.

❐ When a child dies much sympathy is rightly shown to the bereaved parents. When a couple are denied a child because of infertility, the emotional reaction can be similar to the grieving process of bereaved parents. They go through shock, despair, and for some, acceptance, yet there is no funeral to mark the loss and allow mourning to publicly take place. For couples who choose to keep their situation private, there is very little or no support available to them. Even when couples do confide in others, it is difficult for those who have not been through infertility to appreciate the full extent of the emotional pain involved.

❐ There are no simple solutions to this situation. One can only hope that with good counselling, grieving and the passage of years, you will come to live with your situation should a pregnancy not occur. Acceptance and valuing what you have may come in time. Be gentle with yourself, be loving with your partner.

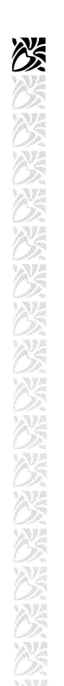

I am adopted, and long to have a child with whom I am biologically related.

❑ There can be a double feeling of sadness for those who are experiencing infertility and who are adopted. Whilst research has shown that most adopted children are happy with their adoptive families, finding out that you are infertile shatters any hopes of being genetically linked for the first time to a loved one, and even the hope of a future generation; thus the shock and frustration of infertility are compounded. It is worth recognising that these can be very powerful emotions for some. Share these thoughts with your partner and those whom you can trust.

❑ For those who are considering assisted conception using donor eggs/sperm, it may help to draw upon your own life experience and recognise that it is possible to form deep and loving relationships with people to whom you are not biologically linked. Think about the reasons why you love your parents; the time, enthusiasm, patience they gave you, in short the love that they gave you, not simply the genetic material. When contemplating using donor eggs/sperm, it is very important that both individuals feel they can love a child with whom only one partner has any genetic connection. If one partner has any doubts then this should be discussed at length. For the interests of the child, treatment should not go ahead unless both partners are really sure of this. One adoptee who had come to terms with his situation, did so by thinking positively about the relationships he already had. It is important to allow yourself time to get over the loss.

How do you go about adopting?

❒ This is a totally different experience to having a child who may be biologically linked with you and therefore must not be seen as a substitute pregnancy.

❒ There are far fewer children available for adoption than there used to be (and even fewer babies), so this too is not a straightforward path. If you are interested in this option then telephone your local social services (Adoptions and Fostering) and ask them how you get on the waiting list. Agencies will normally not consider you if you are undergoing infertility treatment so you need to be sure of your decision.

❒ There are a number of books outlining the stories of couples who have adopted. There are also support groups to talk with other prospective adopters. There is normally a series of sessions introducing people to the adoption process. These are organised by your local Social Services Department or Adoption Agency.

❒ We cannot stress enough how different an experience adoption is. A point to be aware of when going for adoption is that the social workers (who are normally very sensitive) are trying to find a set of parents for children in their care, rather than finding you a child. Be prepared for this change of emphasis, spend time considering what you can offer should you decide to take this option.

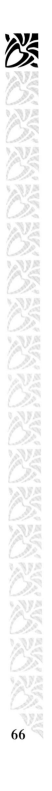

Experiences

The experience of infertility is usually very private. Couples go through different thoughts and feelings at different times. The following experiences have been written by people who were faced with infertility at one time in their lives. These accounts, written in their own words, have been included to help you explore your own feelings and to reassure you that your reactions are similar to those of others faced with infertility problems. The emotional difficulties are overwhelming and, for many sharing their experiences is only possble after they have finished their treatment; to discuss at the time may be too painful.

One noticeable theme is how unprepared we all are for infertility, as from puberty we are advised by parents and teachers how easy it is to get pregnant, and how women particularly must be careful. It is understandable therefore that fertility is something that we take for granted. As more people share their experiences, others will come to realise that infertility affects many families and friends. By raising awareness now, the shock of infertility for future couples may be lessened.

The writers of these accounts have different endings to their experiences. Some have come to terms with the fact that their lives will be childfree; some now have children with whom they are biologically linked; some are families through adoption. You too will resolve your situation in time. Keep a long term perspective of your treatment, this may help you cope with emotional ups and downs of day to day living. Couples have treatment; individuals have feelings; hence these are individuals' experiences.

Philip's Experience

It was a very happy and hopeful day when we first decided to try for a baby. The end of contraception, and now lovemaking seemed to have two purposes - a show of affection, and also our hope of creation.

We carried on trying for a baby for a while but with no success. Why? Time passed, time passed. We reached a point when we thought we'd better see a doctor. We went together but I was referred to the hospital to donate some sperm for tests. The results came back and the doctor raised some concerns. A second test revealed low motility. I worried that it was my fault. I think back now and wish I'd been more assertive. I wanted the results in writing, I wanted an analysis I could understand. How could something be definite from two tests?

Our tests continued and now it involved my partner, humiliating investigations and a laparoscopy operation. I worried for her that day. It seemed I was the cause of her investigations and yet I was helpless.

The results came, still no clear answer. This so called "science" with white coats seemed more and more ad hoc and experimental. We are guinea pigs for them. I still feel responsible, to some degree, for our infertility but how much can I blame myself for the potential limits of my body? It's not my fault . We have tried and tried with still no success, but we are still together.

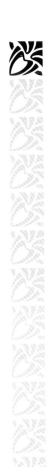

Tracey's Experience

It never occurred to me that having a baby would be a problem. I'd been on the Pill for years and only came off when my first marriage broke up. By the time I remarried I was nearly 30 and my partner was seven years older. We decided we wouldn't wait, we'd have a baby straight away.

But it didn't work out like that. Month after month I cried as we were disappointed yet again. After a year I went to the doctor and was given a chart and thermometer. Six months later we were sent to hospital. Two visits later I'd been seen by three doctors, was sick of being examined and had been told that the chances were that we would have to wait a year for an exploratory operation.

Desperate by that time, and against all our principles we went private. The gynaecologist was wonderful, down to earth, patient and understanding. My partner was tested first. His sperm count was high therefore it felt as though it was my fault. At this point I was tempted to give up, but I knew how important children were to him, and by now I was obsessed "with succeeding." There was pressure also from both sets of parents, neither of whom had any grandchildren.

I was booked in for a D.&C. and a laparoscopy. A week off work so now my colleagues knew. I was hysterical and nearly didn't go. Afterwards my worst fears were confirmed and my tubes were blocked and I wasn't producing eggs on my own.

I will never forget the numbness I felt as I listened to the surgeon, or the pain that followed once the numbness wore off.

Annie's Experience

Children were something I completely took for granted as being part of my future. It never occurred to me, I had never considered that it could be otherwise. I would wait until the time was right, then I would have them, probably two.

The right time came nearly ten years ago. I had just turned thirty. We began to try to conceive. We knew we might wait for some months. A year later we were still waiting, we were beginning to be worried, to fear there may be a problem. Our G.P. agreed to refer us to the local infertility clinic. If we had a problem we would find someone to help us sort it out.

The next three to four years were a bad spell in my life, it's not an exaggeration to say a nightmare. I felt embarrassed and degraded by the investigations, offended and patronised by the doctors. We never did discover why we were not able to produce a child. My partner and I struggled to support each other. Every month the wait, then the pain.

During this time it became difficult to talk to people about children, to be with family and friends with children or to be near pregnant women, especially pregnant friends.

It was difficult to cope with other people's assumptions that we had no children through choice. It felt impossible to talk about, we found it hard to express and others found it hard to hear. I felt damaged, invisible and left out. I knew that having a child was what I wanted most in my life and I could not foresee a future without children. We were all too aware that we were being damaged by the experience of infertility.

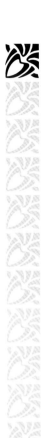

After about four years we decided to stop seeing the doctors, to at least have a break from it. We didn't ever go back, deciding that we'd leave that to fate. We began to explore adoption, a process fraught with difficulties of its own. I began to understand more about the pain we were suffering. I began to allow myself to own and to mourn the two little "ghosts" who seemed so real to me. They are a part of me and that's OK.

People find different ways which are right for them. It is possible to survive infertility.

Coping with bad news.

Psychologists and grief counsellors recognise that as individuals we cope with "bad news" in a variety of different ways, however the following four stages are often a typical pattern that people go through. It may help you to know where you are emotionally and to alleviate some future pain by anticipating what may be ahead for you as a couple.

DISBELIEF OR DENIAL. This initial stage is when you find it difficult to come to terms with information you have been given. We are often in a state of shock, not really being able to take in what has been said.

ANGER AND GUILT. This is when we want to blame somebody, we may feel bitter, there may be emotional outburts directed towards those who are around us e.g. partners, family, doctors.

DEPRESSION. Here we turn inwards and may become isolated. Our relationships may suffer. A sense of loss is experienced and a grieving process starts to take place, slowly this leads to the final stage.

LEARNING TO COPE. By this stage, we start to develop our own ways of dealing with difficult situations relating to our infertility. We may never fully stop hurting from the pain of infertility, but it is possible to reach a sort of acceptance. By choosing to face up to the situation we are taking control and empowering ourselves.

Positives

Infertility is hard to deal with, but out of every bad experience good will come. Reassure yourself with the following positive thoughts:

–you learn about yourself, your partner and the relationship. There is a great possibility of growing and developing together.

–you see life from a different perspective. You know, perhaps more than others, what is really important, you are less likely to be upset by little things.

–you have developed sensitivity and can be more caring towards one another, you become a better listener.

–through honesty you become closer to friends and family, discovering that friendships developed in times of need are strong ones indeed.

–you value the present.

–you realise that children are not a right.

–you have time to think about child rearing and because of this, should you become pregnant you are likely to be very caring parents.

–you learn about life.

Final word

Whatever your situation is with regards to having children, we really hope it gets better.

We cannot control our infertility, but we can control how we see it.

Enjoy your time together and relish the relationships you have.

Keep positive.

Don't be too hard on your self and above all value yourself. You are important whether you have children or not.

We hope this book has shown that those of us faced with infertility share similar feelings and reactions, and that this information will help you to cope and move on emotionally, increasing your confidence and self-esteem.

Glossary

The aim of this book is to explore the emotional side of infertility, but sometimes we feel powerless because we don't understand the language used by the medical profession, or occasionally we may forget parts of what we were told. Your doctor is the best person to explain conditions and treatments to you. The following is a short alphabetical selection of some of the most common words or phrases you may come across whilst undergoing investigations. It is recognised that new treatments may be developed, so always consult your doctor.

Donor insemination A technique using healthy motile sperm from an unknown donor. The sperm is usually placed by a nurse at the neck of the womb, while the woman remains conscious.

Endometriosis Sometimes fragments of the endometrium (lining of the womb) are found outside the uterus affecting the reproductive organs. This can cause infertility in severe cases.

FSH Follicle stimulating hormone causes the follicles to develop each month within the ovary. Follicles contain the eggs.

GIFT Gamete intra-fallopian transfer. The ovaries are stimulated with drugs (gonadotrophins), the eggs collected at laparoscopy, mixed with the sperm and replaced in the tube where fertilization hopefully takes place.

Hysterosalpingogram An x-ray where dye inserted at the cervix shows up any defect in the uterus or obstruction in the tubes.

ICSI Intracytoplasmic sperm injection. Eggs are recovered following gonadotrophin stimulation of the ovaries, as in I.V.F. A single sperm is then injected into each egg to achieve fertilisation.

IVF In vitro fertilisation (literally means fertilised in glass, dish/"test tube"). This can be a natural cycle (no drugs required) but more commonly and successfully a stimulated cycle using gonadotrophins. The eggs are collected through the vagina with the help of ultra sound, fertilised with the sperm in the laboratory and up to three embryos replaced either into the uterus or tube. A general anaesthetic is not required.

LH Luteinising hormone is released in a surge from the pituitary gland at mid-cycle, maturing the egg and triggering ovulation.

Laparoscopy An operation which allows the ovaries, fallopian tubes and the womb to be examined, using an instrument called a laparoscope, which is inserted in the abdomen under general anaesthetic.

Oestrogens Hormones secreted by the ovaries causing the lining of the womb to thicken after menstruation.

Progesterone This hormone, coming from the collapsed follicles maintains the endometrium in a state of readiness for a fertilised egg to implant.

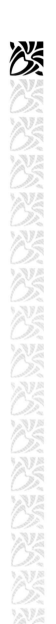

Useful Addresses

CHILD
A self-help charity organisation offering counselling, education and advice for the subfertile
43 St Leonards Road, Bexhill-on Sea, East Sussex.
TN40 1JA
Telephone: 01424 732361

ISSUE
An organisation offering help for childless couples
509 Aldridge Road, Great Barr, Birmingham. B44 8NA
Telephone: 0121 3444414

D.I. NETWORK
A self-help group for those who are considering conception via donor insemination
P.O. Box 265, Sheffield. S3 7YX

RELATE
Offers counselling for those seeking help with relationship difficulties
Herbert Gray College, Little Church Street, Rugby.
CV21 3AP
Telephone: 01788 573241

PARENT TO PARENT INFORMATION SERVICE
An organisation providing help and support for those with any queries concerning adoption
P.P.I.S., Lower Boddington, Daventry, Northants.
NN11 6YB
Telephone: 01327 260295

BRITISH AGENCY FOR ADOPTION AND FOSTERING
11 Southwark St, London SE1 1RQ

Useful Books

Getting Pregnant
Robert Winston

Infertility "WHY US"
Dr A Stanway

Infertility – your questions answered
S. L. Tan and H. S. Jacob

Coping with Childlessness
Diane and Peter Houghton

(All titles above are available from booksellers and ISSUE, formerly the National Association for the Childless, address on previous page).

The Gift of a Child
Robert and Elizabeth Snowden

(available from booksellers or the University of Exeter Press, Streatham Drive, Exeter.)

My Story
A book written to explain donor insemination to a young child

(available through D. I. Network – see facing page)

About the author

This book was written by Chrissie Jones.

Having experienced the difficulties of childlessness first hand, and having listened and talked about infertility with over thirty couples, she has produced this book to help people currently faced with infertility.

Chrissie is a college teacher and graduated from the University of Sheffield in Sociology with Psychology. She has undertaken training in counselling skills and has used all of this to approach the problem of infertility.

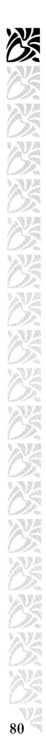